Secrets of a Toddler: Diet, Energy, and Success

I0438491

Laura Andolini

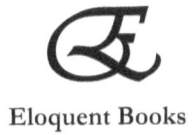

Eloquent Books

Copyright 2010
All rights reserved — Laura Andolini

No part of this book may be reproduced or transmitted in any form
or by any means, graphic, electronic, or mechanical, including
photocopying, recording, taping, or by any information storage
retrieval system, without the permission, in writing, from the
publisher.

Eloquent Books
An imprint of Strategic Book Group
P.O. Box 333
Durham CT 06422
www.StrategicBookGroup.com

ISBN: 978-1-60911-445-9

Printed in the United States of America

To my son Vito

Contents

Foreword

I knew that being a mother was going to change my life, but I never knew that my son would become my greatest teacher. Without verbal language, he silently teaches me about life's simple lessons, and that I forgot how to live a balanced life. He lives only by his feelings and intuition, which is something that I lost as I have grown up. He hasn't had the chance to experience anything that could change his ability to live naturally, or to do and become whatever his thoughts and body tell him to.

As an ACE certified personal trainer, a licensed vocational nurse, and a chef, I thought I knew about a lot of things, until I became a mom. I learned how to live on two hours of sleep and go to work the next day, that cleanliness is overrated, and that all pacifiers are not created equal. I also learned that a young child intuitively eats a very balanced diet, and has a healthy mindset when it comes to food until they discover the adult world of restraints and dieting.

I wish that everyone could experience being a parent, but more so, that the parents already out there could grasp what these kids have to show us. They are the source. They are everything that we lost sight of as we grew up, making them the only way back to normalcy.

Many people who write books and magazines on diets have some type of weight loss success story. I am proud to say that I have the best kind of success story—I have never been fat! I have fluctuated a few pounds here and there, but I have never been overweight. Even when I was pregnant, I only gained nineteen pounds and still had a healthy boy who weighed eight pounds and two ounces. I eat the things that I want to eat and I am on no diet, whatsoever. I exercise regularly and enjoy everything that I eat, as well as everything I do. I actually, enjoy it even more now that I have written this book; only because it put me face to face with what bothered me about food and dieting, and forced me to address those issues head on. This book helped me to ask myself the very questions that I have answered in it, and balance the imbalances that I once had. It has become my purpose to share this with everyone, especially parents who can break the cycle of dieting and obesity. Bon Appetite!

Part I

Diet Secrets of a Toddler

Diet Secrets of a Toddler

The other day I was trying unsuccessfully to get my eighteen-month old son to eat something—anything. I thought, *Wow! If only he could share his secret of how to deny food, we would have the weight loss plan of the century! Can you imagine everyone resisting all of their food temptations and eating only when it is completely necessary? This little man holds the secret to reversing the obesity epidemic and in turn, would decrease the incidence of diabetes, heart disease, cancer, and the list goes on and on. This boy who can't even talk yet could single-handedly resolve the health insurance crisis, if only he could speak! It is my job as his mother to translate his babbles, cries, and scrinchy faces to share his secret with the adults who need it.*

Some of the ideas here might be controversial or seem to go against a healthy diet, but I assure you that it is quite the contrary. The problem that I see with almost every diet is the lack of balance. I don't mean nutritional balance; I mean mental balance. Every day we are bombarded by advertisements, persuasions for different diets, and methods to lose weight; so much so that it makes us so incredibly conscious of food that we lose focus of food's real purpose—to nourish us. Food is not the enemy in our battle of the bulge; our minds are the enemy. If we could only return to the fresh ideas and feelings about food and many other aspects of life that we had as children, we might just live more balanced lives and be thinner, healthier, and happier too.

Many people have asked me how I stay so lean, being a mom with pretty much no time to myself. I answer with, "My son keeps me thin!" People usually think I mean that I have to chase him around all day, which is true, but that is not the reason why he keeps me thin. To avoid the strange looks and lengthy explanations, I smile and nod and never explain exactly what my true thoughts are. That's when I decided to write a book about it.

I'm Too Busy to Eat That!

With ten thousand different things to do every day, it's a wonder how people have time to eat enough to get fat! It is said that one of the top ten reasons that people eat, is boredom. What? How is this possible when people often say they are too busy to cook, eat healthy, and exercise? How is eating food more exciting and fulfilling than taking a walk outside? I'm sure that if you asked a toddler if they preferred to go to the park or to stay home and eat a sandwich, they would choose the park every time. I witnessed a good example of this at the park just the other day. There was a group of young children and toddlers who were attending a birthday party. It came time for them to eat the beautiful, delicious cake that the mother probably slaved over that very morning, and each child received a piece of cake. Some children took a bite or two before one child ran to play with the new toys in the sandbox. Within less than one minute, the children dispersed to go run and play. The poor mother was left with something like twenty pieces of her lovely cake that hadn't even been tasted. Those kids were focused on having a great day, cake or no cake. You can bet that had this been a party for adults there most certainly would have been some people devouring the first piece of cake and returning for seconds. What happens in our minds as we get older that makes food a higher priority than play? Does food become more appealing? Do our lives become so uninteresting that the best part of a party is the cake? It seems as though it is as simple as what was observed at the park—a shift in focus. We become lazy and less and less energetic as we go to school, then work, and think we deserve to sit down at the end of each day and eat whatever we want because the day was so long. We look at food as a means to nurture us because no one else is there to do it anymore. Now *you're* the one baking the cake and you can't understand why someone wouldn't want to eat it. What a *waste!* The tables have turned.

What a WASTE!

Waste not; want not. I definitely *do not* want extra stuff on my waist! And that's exactly what we need to understand, to keep tons of weight off of millions of people. My son taught me something about wasting food. He decided he was finished with his plate of finger food stuff and very abruptly, and with impressive precision, threw the plate and its contents into my lap. He was very satisfied with this gesture, simply because he was not hungry anymore and got rid of the offensive leftovers to move on to the next mess-making task. Have you ever seen a toddler eat something because they didn't want to waste it? No way! They don't care about that stuff! It's us, adults that see a different value in food, which usually has something to do with money or earnings. Let's step back from that for a second. If you eat something that your body doesn't need, isn't that called being excessive? Isn't that somewhat synonymous with *wasteful?* And everyone knows that if we eat more than we need, we get fat. And if we get fat, we become unhealthy and acquire unpleasant illnesses. So what really *is* the value of that food? If you don't benefit from it, and in fact hurt yourself by eating it, it is less of a waste to throw it away than to eat it. The same holds true for eating at restaurants. How many toddlers do you see leaving a restaurant, half in a food coma because they just consumed an entire day's worth of calories in one sitting? I sure haven't seen any. I have seen some throw two day's worth of calories on the floor, though. Of course the best option is to only take what we need, in order to be sure not to waste in any sense; but I'm pretty sure that most of us don't have an exact food meter. Just learn to be conscious of what seems to be a reasonable amount of food and what is excessive. And by all means, when you are not hungry anymore…stop eating! Just don't throw your plate.

Another interesting example of this overeating problem can be observed with the family dog. Dogs still have that primitive idea of scarcity, in their brains, and no conscious mind to fight it. If you give a dog a bowl of food he or she will eat it. If you give a dog two bowls of food, he or she will eat it, and on and on until they are somewhat like the dog version of foie gras. However, if you give the dog one of my sister's vegan cookies he or she will put it under the couch until it stinks (more than it already does). The point here is that we are arguably more reasonable and in control of ourselves than dogs, so let's act like it! Only eat what you need.

Cut Off the Crust or It Goes in the Garbage!

I remember when I was little, if something wasn't *just so,* I wouldn't have anything to do with it. My dad would make me toaster pastries in the morning and I refused to eat it unless he cut off the crust, which he always did, even before I asked. (Thanks, Dad.) I was no exception. Kids are picky. I find now, especially after attending culinary school, that I now am not very picky with food, if at all. What changed? I have no idea. There just really aren't that many flavors and textures that bother me in foods, anymore. This is great for those dinners cooked by friends and family that used to cause food resistance and occasional vomiting, but it is not good for the diet. When we lose our discriminating tastes that we once had as children, any food becomes fair game.

Whether it's those greasy, chemical muffins at the office or mom's meatloaf, the things that used to make you cringe, you now find yourself eating regularly. Less discrimination equals more food to eat.

My son has never, ever *settled* on a certain food just because he was hungry or because it was offered to him. He could be *starving* but if it's not what he wants he will wait until the right food presents itself. (By waiting, I mean screaming like he is being pinched by one hundred crabs.) I explained this concept to one of my friends because it used to drive me crazy that she would treat hunger like it was an emergency. She would eat anything that was around the very second that she would become hungry, and if she didn't eat something all hell would break loose. Needless to say, she was about thirty pounds overweight. Since I was pretty sure that she was in no immediate danger of starvation, I stopped her from eating something she didn't really like and asked her to think about what she was doing (besides freaking out for no reason). I suggested to her that she wait to eat until she had something that she really, really wanted to taste. I told her I would take her to her favorite sandwich shop if she would just relax and listen to me. She agreed and I bought her, her favorite kind of sandwich. While she was eating it I asked her if she was happier waiting to eat this, the taste she truly wanted to experience, than eating a bunch of unsatisfying junk. To my surprise, this really struck a cord and stuck with her and she changed the way she looked at food. Within about three months she had lost ten pounds, just by regaining her discriminating appetite. Wow! Kids are so smart!

The Nonstop Food Clock

Many people these days are on this type of diet where they eat five times a day, or some foolish thing like that. This is a *diet?* Really? I have tried something similar to this and I can tell you that it is absolutely ridiculous. It is true that your metabolism will stay at higher levels when you are constantly trying to digest all of that excess food, but usually the real eating disorder that makes people fat is their mind, not their eating schedule. Let's think about this logically. They say you burn about three hundred extra calories a day by eating every three to four hours, which very likely is true, but how many extra calories do you take in by eating five times a day? Even if your meals are small it is very difficult to stay within your daily caloric range when it is so widely distributed. Not many people have the self-control to eat only eight almonds at a time. The real problem with this constant eating is just that—you're constantly eating! This means that you are thinking about eating all of the time! Isn't that called an eating disorder?

Children don't give a hoot what time it is, where they are, what their plans are for the day and certainly don't plan when they will be hungry or eat around all of those daily activities. They live their lives and let hunger happen; they don't try to prevent it! And then when hunger does happen, they choose just what they want in the correct amount to be satisfied and no more. This is probably the healthiest way of eating that I have ever seen!

Another interesting eating problem that I have seen in someone that I know is an obsession with eating enough fiber. I think this problem might have stemmed from attending nursing school and having to record BMs (bowel movements) in a book. When you have to make notes of other people's bowel irregularities, you suddenly become very conscious of your own. I understand this because I went to nursing school too, but she takes it way past the line of normal. She checks every food item for its fiber content and makes almost all food choices based on this information. I think she read somewhere that fiber can reduce the amount of calories absorbed by the digestive system, which is true, but if you eat all the time and eat extra things with fiber just to stay regular, you are still eating more than you would if you weren't so concerned about your weight and fiber intake. The advice here? Forget about it! Be like the kids! They don't think about their BMs all day or what they have to eat to be regular! Of course, some fiber is very beneficial and I recommend eating whole grains often, just don't get your head so wrapped around it that it dictates everything you eat.

The Weight of the Issue

Many people who are trying to lose weight think that it is a good idea to weigh every food item that they eat, to be absolutely certain that they are consuming the amount of calories that they are aiming for in a day. I have even seen some fancy scales where you can type in the food item to be weighed and it can give you the all of the nutritional information of that particular item right there. This is great if you have some type of health issue that requires you to limit or increase your intake of a certain nutrient, but if you are a healthy, normal person, this is called an eating disorder! It's madness! In my opinion, any time someone is thinking so hard about their eating habits or spending time and money to analyze so precisely what they put in their bodies, this is a major eating disorder. It is also interesting to me that people are really concerned with their metabolism. They eat all day long because it's supposed to raise your metabolism. Hmmm, this sounds fishy…eating for the purpose of being able to eat more. Why not just eat the right amount in the first place and get on with it? I guess I missed something there. When most people think about eating disorders they think of the usual bulimia and anorexia, but if you look into the definition of these diseases, they have a common characteristic: obsession with food and appearance. Weighing food, thinking about food, worrying about food, changing the way you live your life because of your fears of food…these are all signs of eating disorders. Society, commercials, weight loss gimmicks, and fad diets that envelope us every day are creating these eating disorders in millions of people, and instead of making them healthy, it's making them fat. It's creating a food-obsessed nation—a nation of eating disorders. The only way to reverse it is to return to who we once were before all of this diet stuff came into our lives. We can bring back these easier, simpler, and more balanced ways of living by observing those who are living it now—kids! When we are searching for anything we usually have to go back to the source. Our source as humans, is children. Explore that and you'll be amazed at what you'll uncover.

That's Not Food!

Today I made some baby potatoes and set them aside to cool. When they were cooled off I was preparing to make some potato salad. At this time, my son walked over to me in the kitchen and did the leg grab that toddlers try to melt their parents with before or after they do or did something that they shouldn't have. I thought that he might like to try a potato that was just his size so I handed him one, thinking that this could be something he might actually eat. He examined it thoroughly and proceeded to stick that little, bitty finger all the way through it and then throw it on the floor. It hit the ground with an amusing *thunk* and he laughed a deep-bellied laugh and did it again. He didn't even view the potato as a food item. How interesting! Toddlers are still learning to identify what food even is, let alone its effects on the body or what a diet is. They have not yet acquired this preoccupation with food that so many adults have.

If you didn't even know what a diet is, would you think about food as much as you do? I know that I wouldn't. I never cared about food or diets and I was always very thin. It wasn't until I became aware of diets and the desire of many girls to be thin that I even gained a pound. I gained weight only after I started to pay attention to what I was eating and became fearful of becoming fat. It is important to understand that food is good for you when you eat the right things at the right times. There should never be guilt associated with eating, because it is a necessity of life! It should be invigorating! We need not to teach about diets, but about nutrition and how to feel good about eating, instead of how to restrain ourselves. You shouldn't have to make the right *choices* when it comes to food because we should be taught that some things just aren't food. Donuts, things full of dyes and chemicals, overly processed nasti-ness—these things are simply not food. This is called pica. Pica is the desire to consume non-food items like clay, dirt, paint chips, etc. Pica is usually the result of malnutrition and lack of nutrients, and so the body's emergency response system tells you to eat weird stuff. When the body then thinks that it received nutrition through this consumption of non-food items, it still feels that the job was done, and will prompt you to eat it again. Eating junk food is no different. The body thinks that it was provided with what it needed, but actually wasn't, and it wants more junk. Donuts, sugary foods, and foods with chemicals are not nutritious and serve no purpose for us. After I pondered this idea for a while, I found it strange how unfood-like many things people eat today, really are. If a child was never told that processed fruit snacks were food, they would probably never even identify them as such. It is now our job to only introduce true food items to our growing members of society and stop the junk food and diet cycle.

Taste It before You Swallow

Anton Ego, in the children's movie *Ratatouille,* was a mean food critic who was getting ready to eat at the restaurant where the rat worked. Chef Linguini told Mr. Ego that he was "thin for someone who liked food," to which, Mr. Ego responded, "I don't like food; I love it! If I don't love it, I don't SWALLOW!" A very intriguing concept that was addressed briefly when we discussed how children are so picky about food. They truly *taste* the food. Many times even I have wolfed some food down because I was in a hurry to do something else and barely even tasted what I ate. It didn't matter if it was a succulent piece of cake or liver and onions, the way that it was just choked down! When we don't give ourselves the time to really taste the food and feel joyous about it, our brains really miss out on that chemical change that creates happiness and satisfaction. This makes our brains say, "Hey, what happened? I missed it! Do it again!" And later on, you will give in to that and eat more. When you put something in your mouth; taste it! This moment of enjoyment is a gift! Don't ruin what the food is trying to offer you; take an extra few minutes to pay attention to what you are doing. Your body will thank you later by not expanding.

It has been said already that when kids don't like something, they don't eat it. That means that they always follow the "taste before you swallow," rule. Adults tend to stay on autopilot throughout most of the day. We are stuck in ruts of getting things done, whether it's work, eating, doing yard work, watching the kids, or sitting around. We often find ourselves doing things just because that's what we always do. Often times, it doesn't even occur to us to pay attention to the details, like what our food tastes like. We make something and eat it because eating is on the list of things to do, or because of the many other reasons why people eat when they actually aren't even hungry. If we could just slow down and follow this simple rule, we might look more like Anton Ego.

What Did You Just Say!

It is impossible to teach a very young child everything they need to know to be polite. They just don't have that filter yet that tells them not to say and do certain things. On numerous occasions, I have witnessed (or personally experienced) a child embarrassing the daylights out of an adult by saying something that is impolite, but always the absolute truth. My dad once told me a story about when he was five years old and he told his aunt that she was fat. He said that his mom was mortified and he was in big trouble. He still feels bad about it, to this day. Why should he feel bad? He just made an honest and true observation. It wasn't even in his awareness that fat was offensive, or even how people get fat in the first place. It's funny that kids can point out our sorest of insecurities at the worst of times. The interesting thing is that as adults we should be aware of what insecurity actually is. Wikipedia says a person who is insecure lacks confidence in their own value and capability. This means there is something wrong with *that* person; not the one who says something about the insecurity. If someone is insecure about being fat, there is clearly an imbalance there. My motto for this is, "If you can be embarrassed by the truth, you need change in your life." If you have something so obviously wrong or different about you that you can be humiliated by a child pointing it out, that's something you should probably take care of. Children do need to be taught proper manners, but equally, we need to teach ourselves to recognize the most obvious of our own problems and confront them like the adults that we think we are.

Food Generations

Food can be a great pleasure in life that we get to enjoy everyday. This is why overeating has become such a widespread problem. It wasn't that long ago, certainly still in my parents' time, when food was prepared everyday by someone—usually a mom. I know a lot of moms today who don't know how to turn on the stove. Microwaves, fast food, and takeout have replaced a very important part of the enjoyment of food. Memories are often made by the smells and tastes of food that can take us back to a different time and place. I can remember very vividly, the taste of my grandma's food and the cookies that she made and stashed for me during Christmas, because she knew they were my favorite. Smell and taste are the senses that are the most associated with memory. I would hate to think of this generation of children growing up with non-cooking moms to be brought back to their childhood years from now by the smell of a fast food burger with fries or those cinnamon buns at the mall. Also, when food is prepared by someone or better yet, with someone who we care about, that food becomes nourishment in more than the physical sense. I have seen a grown man cry over a dish that tasted just like his mother used to make, but I have never seen someone sobbing over a plate of chicken fingers at a chain restaurant.

Holidays are often a reason to chow down on some tasty, yet sometimes unhealthy foods. At Christmas we are bombarded by cookies, cakes, ham, candies, pies, etc. I have heard of people gaining upwards of seven pounds during the holiday season! Holy smokes! Just to put that into perspective that is 24,500 extra calories in a matter of weeks! That is disgusting! I would have to try pretty hard to do that to myself. That is a perfect example of not appreciating the food for what it is—nourishment created with love and care! It's something to be respected and appreciated not stuffed into our bodies until we feel sick! If you truly value that food, you take what you need, enjoy it, and feel grateful for it. Not to mention, feel better about yourself and healthy. I enjoy watching children during these holidays because they really take it all for what it is. They bake the cookies with their families, build gingerbread houses, and enjoy the candy in their stocking; usually only after the playing and construction are finished. The food is an activity in itself and sometimes not even eaten. I have made gingerbread houses that are probably still lying around, petrified in a storage unit somewhere. I was so proud of what I had made that it would have been a disgrace to destroy it just to eat it! The food revolves around the holiday, not the other way around. Also, these times of sweets and abundance of food only come around a few times a year, so one or two treats for celebration won't hurt anybody. It's when we overdo it and lose that sense of specialness that should be associated with that food that we have erred. I think that every child has overdone it on candy and other foods once or twice, but most times that's all it takes. They usually remember that sick feeling and take it easy the next time. Apparently, adults have short term memory loss pretty frequently because I see even my own family members stuff themselves to sickness at many gatherings. We need to set a better example than that!

I have now decided to make it a priority to be sure that I provide my son with these fulfilling experiences with food and to make sure that he understands the traditional and cultural reasons for cooking and eating certain things. When we can attach food to something greater than just something to scarf down because that's what we know how to do, we naturally pace ourselves while eating; appreciating what it is, who made it, and where it came from. The diet here is simple appreciation and conservation of something sacred to us.

Warning! Consult Your Physician

Today, while I was on one of the machines at the gym, I noticed the warning sticker that is on many pieces of equipment at the gym, stating that anyone who is going to begin an exercise regimen should consult a physician. As a personal trainer myself, I know that the clients of trainers often need to have a physical exam by a doctor before they can begin an exercise program. What about all of the people who sit on the couch all day, or at their desks without a chance to move around? Shouldn't they need a physical to see if they can stand the risks of sitting around all day? Shouldn't someone give them some type of order to at least get up and walk around a few times a day? We know the risks of a sedentary lifestyle greatly outweigh any benefit, and vice versa for exercising. It seems to me that we have some things backwards here.

I learned in a few different ways after becoming a mother that exercise is a privilege. I used to dread going to the gym everyday and just did it because I would feel bad if I didn't do it. Now I am lucky to have the chance to go to the gym two or three times per week and I look forward very much to that time to myself! I pack more into that hour at the gym than I used to get out of three hours before, and I enjoy every minute of it! It is some of the only time that I have to myself, and I can even watch TV shows that don't start with *Meeska, Mooska,* or *Mickey Mouse!* I can't wait to go and get my workout in so I can feel better about the rest of my day and relax, not to mention, being in better shape to chase around a toddler!

A child does not have the capability of sitting around all day. It is just not how they are made. Grade school with no recess would be an absolute disaster. What we consider to be exercise, they consider play or free time. They wait all day in school just to go outside and let it all out. If you ask a kid what they want for their birthday they will often say that they would like a bicycle. I know some women who would find it insulting to receive a bicycle as a gift, like it's the equivalent of someone calling them fat. What changes in us as we age? Why does exercise become a chore instead of the privilege that it once was? After I asked myself this question, I realized that I was, at times, guilty of this very change myself. I felt ashamed that I had lost my zest for getting out and exploring, playing, and *living*. It was a life-changing mind alteration. Now I can't stand to sit too long, and I can't with a toddler around, anyway! He will fuss all day until I take him outside to play. He keeps me balanced and reminds me to keep doing things, and not to lose momentum as life goes on.

Health is also a privilege. There are millions of people born into this world, unhealthy; without even being given the chance to experience a healthy body. Health is a generous gift that should be taken care of. If someone gave you a Ferrari, would you drive it through a field of mud and rocks, or neglect washing or waxing it until it became worn out, dirty, and ugly? Would you put regular or premium gas in the tank? Our bodies are much more precious than a Ferrari and yet we fail to do basic maintenance on them for years and years, or put bad fuel in them and wonder why there are so many chronic illnesses occurring at exponentially increasing rates.

But My Dad Said...

Children think that their parents are always right. To children, parents are an entirely different species that are bigger and know all kinds of stuff without ever having to learn it. Parents are Wikipedia, chefs, musicians, hair stylists, magicians, plumbers, and teachers all in one person. My family and I have many jokes about how we believed everything my dad said, only to find out many years later that he was just joking with us. We would tell our friends about the outlandish things that my dad said were truths, when in fact he was just humoring us. Thanks, Dad.

With that said, children follow what their parents do because to them, parents are always right. If mom eats greasy hamburgers, fried chicken, and food from a box then that's the good thing to eat; right? They think that mom only does things that are good for her and her family, so this must be the right thing to do. Fixing this problem is as easy as taking care of ourselves. Teaching our kids by example how to eat and be healthy can benefit everyone for generations. Parents will learn to be healthier, to take better care of their children, and to be more fun and energetic; and children will have no choice but to learn healthy habits. We only know what we are taught. If we don't want our children to use dirty language, we have to watch our mouths so they never even hear the words. If we want them to eat healthy foods, we have to watch our mouths to make sure only healthy foods enter them.

European Kids Aren't Fat

My son is half French, but that's beside the point here; it just makes for a snappy title. I have spent a lot of time in France and other parts of Europe, learning about food and working as a chef. I can tell you that there are not very many fat people, and almost no obese people in Europe. This seems to be strange because the food there is so tasty and they very rarely use or even sell low-fat or fat-free products. The cheeses, olive oils, fresh breads, and bakery products are everywhere and people eat them every day, just as they have for hundreds of years. In the United States we are told to avoid each one of those products, yet the people in Europe are thinner and healthier than Americans, by far. I hear over and over again that the reason for this result is that Europeans eat everything in moderation. If this is true, then we need to ask why it is so. What is different in their thinking process that makes them eat only what they need to eat? From my observation, there is one very clear difference which relates very much to how they value their food. Europe is much older than the United States; therefore, they have many more traditions with regards to food than we do. They have had traditions in cheese, wine, bread, oil, and other food making for centuries. Many people feel that France has some of the best food in the world, and it is interesting that almost none of it is mass produced as it is in the United States. A European person can most likely tell you not only what the best local cheese is, but where the cheese maker actually lives! I know many Americans who would think of a cheese maker as a cow-poo scooping redneck, but I'm sure that they know someone who works for some large manufacturer or fast food place that produces those non-food items. When you know where your food comes from and the traditions that have been carried out for centuries to create that food, it is natural to put a pretty high value on it. The food is valued, tastes delightful and satisfying, is eaten slowly, and enjoyed for what it is. This is the process, which we need to follow. Attach meaning to the food, eat it, enjoy it, feel satisfied and grateful, and move on. That is one of the differences that I believe European culture has, regarding eating.

When I was living in France, I was surprised by how many businesses still close for midi, the two-hour lunch break between 12:00 P.M. and 2:00 P.M. This meal time is so important that it is necessary to take a two hour break for it! They slow down, prepare their food, eat it slowly, taste it, and enjoy it. They take time to spend with their family and friends in the middle of a busy day, to relax and enjoy some good food together. Then they return to work refreshed and unhurried, which makes for happier workers who work more efficiently. When people are given time to themselves every-day, they don't feel the need to rush through work just to get home. It also keeps the enjoyment in the food; keeping its value so they appreciate it and don't over eat! I know that in the United States we are often pressed for time during lunch, if there is a break at all. I conducted a small experiment to see how fast I could eat a sandwich, just to see if it would be possible to slow it down a bit to enjoy it more. How long did it take me to eat it? Three minutes and forty-seven seconds! I know a lot of people that spend more time than that during a bathroom break! I found that sitting down to relax and enjoy the same kind of sandwich for just ten minutes longer created a much greater feeling of satisfaction and fulfillment; an amount of time I think that we can all find to eat, during the day.

If you go to a restaurant in Europe, don't expect to get a doggy bag at the end of your dinner. They don't serve the monstrous portions that we are familiar with in restaurants here in the U.S. Even after a four-course meal in Europe it is usually still possible to leave the restaurant without a wheelchair; and the best part is that you usually have to walk back home or to the hotel. The chefs in Europe actually *cook* the food you eat too, so again there is that added value to your meal. A small, tasty, fancy dish plated by a professional who clearly created something that you can't make by yourself is valued much higher than a sixteen ounce steak at a chain restaurant. The steak is obviously more food, but as human beings and not animals who are not on a hunt, the fancy dish is a much greater pleasure and an experience. Many chain restaurants in the United States order pre-made food, heat it up, and put it on a plate for you. If you doubt me, go to one of those giant wholesalers that sell food in bulk. Look at the frozen ravioli, bread, pasta sauce, or French fries and see if it looks familiar. I have personally toured some of these warehouses only for professionals and I can tell you that many items, especially desserts like cakes, ice creams, and even cannoli shells are bought by restaurants, pre-made and sold to you at ten times the price without the work. I haven't seen the same type of chain restaurants in Europe and in fact, a few cities protested having McDonald's by throwing rocks through the windows and setting the place on fire! Still want to eat out this weekend? Many small restaurants take pride in buying and cooking their own food. You just have to look around, or use your nose. If it doesn't smell like deep fried food or burnt garlic, try it out.

My son ate his first solid food here in the States. It was Roquefort cheese. Really. He loved it! And later on in his life we tried to give him a slice of the orange cheddar cheese that Americans know so well. To our surprise, he didn't eat it. He didn't even recognize it as food. He will eat parmesan cheese from Parma, but not a U.S. made mozzarella. He will eat a crunchy, fresh baguette, but not a piece of processed white bread. I was almost kicking myself for starting him off on such a pungent food because now he won't eat anything that the rest of the kids here eat! Then I realized that this is a great thing! My son does not have pica! I have taught him about real food and he learned to appreciate it! Wow, this stuff really works!

Doggy Bag

The purpose of this book is to bring us back to who we once were before we ever had the chance to be thrown off track by outside forces. Events and people in our lives shape us every day, making it so very important to always remember who we once were. Childhood is a benchmark to reflect upon to see if we have deviated from where we should be and to gauge our level of happiness. If you feel ashamed of how you have changed, it is never too late to look at that benchmark to see how you can return to a state where you were more pure and unaffected. We are born with our own minds and somehow we let too many things pass our mental filter, altering who we truly are. We often think that we need to be someone different or better; whether at work, in our families, or in our outer appearance. The thing to take from this book is simplicity. Leave things just as they should be. That means remembering how you were supposed to be before other things were allowed to complicate your being. Be grateful for your ability to do and create anything that you want; most importantly yourself.

Part II

Energy and Success

Introduction

Any parent or caretaker of a child could probably say that they have a memory bank full of moments of being amazed and dazzled by what small children can accomplish as they grow and learn. In my own daily struggles to find more energy, success, wisdom, and happiness, I realized that if I just observed my son (twenty-one months old at the moment) and the pathways he follows to learn and expand his abilities exponentially each and every day, that maybe his learning skills could help me to grow and succeed in some aspects of my own life.

His openness to share his emotions and his ease in carrying on about his day inspired me to discover what the true differences are between adults and children, and how they can help us to rediscover what we might have lost along the way, like our resiliency and ability to be who we want to be and do the things that we truly want to do—not what we *think* we *should* do. Before we try to make ourselves important and accepted, we have no need to categorize people, things, and events, leaving an open field for creating and becoming anything, without boundaries.

Countless times my son has laughed at me while I steamed in fury over messes, or frustratedly asked someone who doesn't speak yet why he won't listen to me. I knew then that he must know something that I didn't. It was time to give the parent a lesson.

Many forces enter our lives as we grow older, burying our natural ways of learning and succeeding. When we are young, without so much as language to set our boundaries and limitations, it was natural for us to follow what resonated with us and find success without too much resistance. Those things that didn't serve our contentment were simply denied our attention, although sometimes with the resistance of things like…parents. Now I am the parent, and it is very interesting to regain the natural flow of my being, with the help of my teacher and small friend, my son. He has indeed redirected me to the path that led me to seek out and achieve my goals and purpose in life with greater success than I would have had on my own.

One major obstacle on the road to success is a lack of energy. One will never find success without energy and motivation. I can say that as a parent I need all the energy that I can get! I was reminded of this lack of energy once again this morning, when I was awoken by the sensation of a foreign object being slowly pushed into my eye socket, followed by the squeaky sound of a smiling toddler amusedly sucking away at a pacifier. I am reminded every morning in this manner, consumed with love, that I am indeed the mother of a toddler. As painful, tiring, and trying as it can be at times, I wouldn't have it any other way. If there were just one request that could be fulfilled by my smallest and best friend, it would simply be for him to share his energy with me.

I have been waking up one to three times per night for almost two years now. I never knew that it would be possible to be this tired and still function! I am now more punctual and efficient than I was pre-baby, since the fatigue has taught me new tricks, like how to balance myself just right in order to take a quick nap while standing in line at the bank. I can now take a complete shower in less than ten minutes and clean the bathroom in the time I need to swish my mouthwash. Although some people envied my standing nap trick, I still found myself in an overtired, zombie-like state on most days and wishing only one thing: to have at least the same amount of energy as my son (but even more would be miraculous).

The time had come to figure out how this tiny person could possibly have enough energy to wear me out at the very thought of another sleepless night, followed by a day when I drink endless cups of coffee and implement various energizing techniques just to make it to lunch time. It was necessary to discover how in the world he could possibly be surviving on milk and three-hour intervals of sleep for his entire life thus far. I needed to unveil his secrets in order to take proper care of him and play with him the way that moms should be able to.

I achieved success in my search for energy by observing my son and Zen master, a person who has been untouched by the stresses of the opinions and expectations of others and the monotony and negativity of adult life as most of us know it. I found myself becoming more energized, productive, happy, and successful.

Act As If You Know Nothing— Because Most of the Time It's True

In my pre-parent days I was just like most people I know: I would be engaged in a conversation, having no knowledge about the topic under discussion, but pretending very well that I knew all of the details. I'd play it off until I could go home and look it up on the Internet in case the subject ever came up again. The reality is that most people wouldn't really care if I was uninformed about numerous topics that no one cares about anyway, but it seems to be human nature to not want to feel like an idiot.

I often buy my son a new toy or book and offer a brief demonstration on what you are supposed to do with it. The usual response is a deer-in-headlights "Mom, you're crazy" look, followed by the toy being launched across the room or the book being ripped in half in a satisfied manner, as if to say, "Ah-ha! I have ridded us of the object making Mom weird!" Then he playfully returns to his other toys that have not been tainted by my demonstrations—the ones that he has learned to play with by himself.

It seems that as adults we feel that we have the knowledge and skills necessary to teach the younger generation, like how to live and how to learn things. Just because we have been around longer and done more things does not mean that we did them the right way! Most of our learning comes from categorizing things as good and bad, safe and not safe, light and dark, happy and sad, right and wrong, and on and on. I can say for myself that I am sure that at least a few things have been mixed up in my categorizing process. Some of the documents that should have been filed under "bad" went under "good" and some that went to "should dos" went to "didn't dos," and too many other mix-ups to mention. In most cases it all boils down to trying to file everything in the right order so that other people will accept us and, if we are lucky, even think that we are above average in some way.

I'm not sure that I have ever met a toddler who cared about impressing others with his knowledge; by not worrying about their intellectual image, toddlers open themselves up to learn anything and everything around them, unreservedly. Everything is viewed as fresh, new, interesting, and valid. They have little to no discrimination as to what they will and will not learn. Adults have the unfortunate tendency to categorize everything, even the things that they will learn, into files like: this is for girls, this is for boys; this is for weirdos, people smarter than me, people of a different race or culture, dummies, Republicans, etc. This categorization repels people from something that they might have enjoyed immensely or been very good at.

Most of this preemptive rejection is a result of our need to feel accepted by others. We are made to believe at an early age and in many ways that the most important thing in life is to, well, be important. Being important usually means something like being successful in school and then holding an important title in an important profession. School and work are certainly very important, and merit our best efforts. The problem comes in when one chooses a subject of study or a profession not out of passion and pleasure, but because it is judged as important by others.

Doctors are vital to humans. They are respected and very, very important people, but I know a lot of doctors who are very successful in their practice but very unhappy, because they really wanted to be a hot air balloon pilot or winemaker, teacher, writer, chef, or whatever. When asked why they chose to be doctors, the usual response is something like, "I wanted to help people," or "Doctors make a lot of money," or "My dad told me that this is a good thing to do."

It seems that for small children "important" carries a different meaning. "Important" is synonymous with "I want" or "I like," and somehow they always manage to seek out and obtain whatever it is that they like and want, despite another person's grand efforts to make them do something else.

Back to the toy situation. I have bought my son many, many toys that he didn't like, many of which I thought would be good for his intellectual development, so of course I feared that he would not be as smart as the children who do play with all of those "learning" toys and tools. He was much more content to go outside to observe his surroundings and play with rocks and sticks and stuff. He surprised me with his impressive rock-stacking skills, which required much more balancing techniques and precision than those colorful blocks that I was so upset that he rejected. It was as if he said, "Thanks but no thanks, Mom. Even though I am a baby I can choose the things that I like to play with. Thanks anyway. Oh, and by the way, I'm smarter than you thought I was when you bought me that stupid thing that plays those stupid songs and mocks me." So I learned my lesson and let him be, to make his own decisions and grow in the ways that he feels best.

Anyway, what was I supposed to do? Force him to play with some "educational" thingy just because I bought it and some adults created it thinking that it was important for his intellectual growth? Had I done so, the results would have been disastrous. It would have ended with my son screaming and crying in what would actually amount to an abusive situation. I believe that any time an adult makes a child cry for a foolish reason that it is abuse, so this situation falls under that category.

Now, relating this to adults, should we force ourselves to do things that we don't want to do and fight our way through it, screaming and crying (okay, not screaming and crying, just complaining and getting sick all the time) when we would excel at something else that we enjoy, maybe even be the best at it simply because we enjoy it so much and do it well? With the thousands of opportunities that we have to do and be whatever we want, how does it happen that most people seem to choose something that they don't like? Then they just keep on doing it anyway, even when they *know* that they would be happier and more successful doing something else?

The definition of insanity is doing the same thing over and over but expecting something different to happen. If you hate your job or your choice in education, then do something else. Most people feel that the time spent on that decision or path would be a waste if they decided to make a change. It is important to keep in mind that the time spent was an opportunity to recognize one thing that you definitely do not want to do. I went through nursing school knowing that I didn't want to be a nurse, but I didn't want to feel that I had wasted the time and money going to college for something that I would never use. Currently, I am not a nurse, but I have used my nursing knowledge in many different situations. I value knowing about how to take care of other people and myself, and I do not feel like it was a waste at all. While I was in school, I felt panicked, like I had to finish out the education and work in a field that I would have dreaded for the rest of my life. I have a greater respect for nurses now, knowing what they do, but I want something different. I had to step away and actually start doing something else before I realized how grateful I was for having changed my path. I don't know where I would be if I had stayed with nursing, but I certainly would have missed out on a slew of opportunities and experiences and, of course, finding the things that make me happy and the work that I am good at. Thank you to all of the nurses who do the job because they love it!

Disclaimer!

Now, I'm *not* saying that everyone should quit their jobs or follow some frivolous path in life, or that life is a vacation. To put it simply, if we could follow our instincts as well as children, we might find ourselves happier in many aspects of life, our professional lives included. It is crucial to do well and work hard at school and our jobs throughout our lives, but we need to pay very close attention to the things that we are naturally drawn to, and also to the things that are drawn to us. I have heard many people say that one is "lucky" to do what they love to do for a living, but we *all* are good at something that we love, and we don't all love the same things! There is something for everyone and everyone, with their different desires and talents, should be able to find their "something." If they do, I'm pretty sure that the world would keep on turning around. Maybe even more harmoniously.

In his book, *The Pilgrimage,* novelist Paulo Coelho describes when his guide Petrus taught him about the need to allow change into life: "I must not be afraid to change my life. If I liked what I was doing, very well. But if I did not, there was always the time for a change. If I allowed change to occur, I would be transforming myself into a fertile field and allowing the Creative Imagination to sow its seeds in me... Often people have to accept the changes that destiny forces upon them, but that's not what I'm talking about. I am speaking of an act of will, a concrete desire to battle against everything that is unsatisfying in one's everyday life."

Know When to Walk Away (and Maybe Come Back Later)

My son has returned to the building blocks that he previously rejected. It turns out that after learning with his "natural" rock blocks outside, he wanted the more professional look of hand-crafted, colorful, building blocks. With all of that practice stacking the more difficult rocks outside, he found much pleasure in the ease of stacking geometric figures. One on top of the other, higher and higher they went. Incredible! I would have never believed that my little guy could have such talent at this age! Those blocks that he once angrily knocked over and threw behind the television he now finds great pleasure in stacking and forming into beautiful sculptures! He just wasn't ready for it before he discovered his stacking abilities with the rocks in the yard. Now, when I find his toys laying around that he hasn't played with in a while, I don't give them away like I used to, I save them for a later date when some event or change of mind draws him back to them. We should never give away our possessions and knowledge, because they might be treasures later on!

It seems that almost everything that we do ends up being something that we didn't intend or something unexpected. Things that we thought we didn't like at one point in time often reintroduce themselves in different ways after we have learned about them in different aspects. Things that seemed to frustrate us at one point in time can later become something we fully understand, and even appreciate and enjoy. I used to hate cooking and eating many foods until I traveled and learned about the cultural relevance of food and how it makes up a large part of history, traditions, and the simple joys of everyday life. I continued to learn about food in culinary school and eventually became a chef. This is a great example of doing something else when your current position doesn't put you in the right flow of life. I went from nurse to chef pretty quickly and changed my life from one of misery and discontentment to one of much joy and fulfillment. My nursing skills also came in handy many times in a kitchen full of hot things and sharp objects.

Knowledge Is Cumulative...and Permanent

The other day, we were staying in a hotel room that had a desk positioned just next to a higher table with a television, coffeemaker, and coffee condiments on it. My son was immediately drawn to the desk chair, which had wheels on it, and he wanted to stand on it. He put his hands on the seat and made the chair spin around, but found it difficult to get up onto it. He then discovered that he could push the chair against the desk to make it stop moving. From the chair, he found his way onto the desk, and finally onto the taller table where the coffee condiments were. With full concentration he proudly showed me how much he really does pay attention to every move that I make, when he tore open the coffee and dumped it into the coffee maker—the back part where the water goes, not the correct coffee spot (but still impressive!). Then, he found the sugar packets and put them in his mouth until they were soggy enough to let the sugar out, making for a sweet treat. High on sugar and satisfied with his discoveries, he wanted to return to the floor, but he had pushed the chair away during his ascent. Now the adventure was over, but the return path had been destroyed—there was no way back.

While most people, as they age, fight degenerative diseases that hide our memories somewhere, we never stop to realize that we do indeed remember so, so much. We learn so many things every second of every day, I wonder sometimes whether our focus on what is lost will cause us to keep losing more. If we focus on learning and remembering instead, we'll succeed—it's bound to happen! Our past got us to where we are now, for better or for worse. Like my son, I have been stuck on a high table with no way back down because I had pushed the chair away on the way up. When it's all said and done, memories are what we have left of our lives, friends, experiences, and knowledge. It is important to carefully assess all situations in life and to strategize our movements through life so we don't get stuck in the end, realizing that we forgot something or someone very important along the way. Each decision that we make is a permanent one, and although some decisions can be changed later on to create a different outcome, the path to get there was different so the end result was still affected, sometimes for the better and sometimes for the worse. Either way, it is important to remember every bump and smooth spot along the way and what we learned from everything and everyone for the next time.

If You Don't Get Dirty, You Accomplish Nothing Except Staying Clean

My son was looking dashing in his new jeans and clean, brilliant polo shirt. The sun had just cleared away all of the rain clouds and was drying up the morning showers, making it a lovely day to walk to the park. Upon arrival my son decided to head directly for the wet sandbox and muddy toys. He picked up a muddy rake that someone had left behind and keenly observed that it was far too dirty to use. Naturally, he needed something very clean to wipe it off on—like his brand new polo shirt. And just like that, in a matter of seconds, the fancy, clean shirt was turned into mud clothes. Satisfied with his new treasure of a rake, he could now play contentedly in the sand without having a mucky hand. While digging, he encountered a snail scooting along, trying like hell to get out of harm's way (a two-year-old's grasp). The snail's escape failed and he was scooped up into a tiny hand and shmushed with a proportionately tiny finger. The carcass was jammed into the 2T-sized jean pockets and sealed with a slap. My son decided that the slime from the snail required a rinse from the shooting water fountain that he runs through on hot days. Now dirty, soaked, and sleepy from playing and getting wet, the trip was complete and nap time was next on the list of things to do. Had he been worried about staying clean, he would have never found a rake, learned not to kill snails or other outside critters, or played joyfully in the fountain. He also would have missed his nap time and I would not have gotten anything done around the house.

As we get older it seems that it is more important to keep ourselves and our belongings clean than to just dive into the day and do everything that we can. Looking presentable is mostly important for things like first interviews and dates, just to show that we are pretty and tidy. After the initial meeting, what's more important is what else you have to show besides your fashion sense. Girls are not put here to sit around and look pretty. We are put here to be pretty and also to show that we are good at…everything.

Overstep the
Boundaries

Injury avoidance is also an important part of playing, but we cannot let it ruin our games and progression in life. My son used to really enjoy bending over to scoop water out of the swimming pool with a measuring cup, scaring me half to death every time he did it. I knew one time he was going to fall in, but there was no way to make him understand that it could be fatal. One day, I let him fall in. I was there, of course, to catch him and keep him safe, but he definitely got the idea that the water was scary and dangerous if he was not careful. To my surprise, he never did it again. Everyone knows that experience will teach you more things faster and more permanently than any other method of learning. When we injure ourselves physically or mentally, as long as we can recover, we will raise our awareness and threshold for life's upcoming events. The old saying that whatever doesn't kill you only makes you stronger is valid.

We must occasionally overstep our boundaries in order to see the things that we must be very careful doing, and what we will progress at, given the proper training and practice. We can judge when something is worth the risk and when it is time to find something else to do. Sometimes standing still is the biggest danger of all—if you stand in the street too long, eventually you will be run over. Until the car comes... game on!

There is a strong desire to keep our kids safe and out of trouble, but we need to do so mindfully. We rationalize much of this "watching out" for them as being good for them, when it is actually more for ourselves as parents. We need to know that at least if something happens, we told them so. Concern for safety is very, very important, but it becomes counterproductive when overdone.

"No" is the first word of many children for the obvious reason that they hear it over and over again. It's sad that the first word is often one of negativity. It implies that they feel they *can't* do more things than they *can* do. I often need to tell my son "no," but I make sure that he is redirected and presented with a "yes" situation. The Law of Opposites only works in our favor when we are willing to find the counter-point. If a child is painting the wall with their peanut butter and jelly sandwich, let them know that it is not right, but then turn their attention to a book or toy, or go outside. To stay balanced, the "no" must be replaced with a "yes." Everything is sort of like a modified push-up. It is an exer-cise that is done with the intention of one day becoming strong enough to do the unmodified one. The modified push-up feels close to the real thing, close enough that the transi-tion will be easy when the time comes. It would not be effective to teach someone how to do a sit-up in order to one day do a push-up.

Immunity without Injections

While my son was playing gleefully in the mud he decided to see if what looks like chocolate tastes like chocolate. The answer was not what he had hoped for, but a mom nearby shrieked in terror—like I let my kid eat enriched uranium or something. Most moms get over that "germ freak" thing when something happens like the pacifier falls on the floor at the grocery store, and there is no sink around to rinse it off but the kid is screaming bloody murder so you stick it in their mouth anyway and hope for the best. And sure enough, nothing happened. The baby didn't die of dysentery or contract the flesh-eating virus. Not even a sniffle. These days, people are starting to tell us to wash our hands with regular soap and not antibacterial soap because it is making germs with super strength. All of that resistance against those tiny bacteria and viruses has caused an uproar with vaccines and antibiotics that are becoming ineffective. My dad always said, "You have to eat a pound of dirt before you die," which I think just means that we need to live *with* the dirt, not *against* the dirt. The best way to fight the battle of the germs is to learn to live with them and get sick every once in a while.

Taking a trip to see my family requires taking at least two flights to get there and fighting the freezing, tundra-like environment known as the Midwest. It is quite a circus act to change a squirmy toddler's diaper in a cramped airplane bathroom, and had I gained a few pounds it would have become an impossibility. Then there is the fight in the bathroom when I try my best to do what I need to do and keep the little guy from touching everything and putting his pacifier in that little garbage can of unmentionables.

Of course, by our return home we were all bogged down and fussy with cold and flu symptoms, including my son. He was surprisingly active despite his ailment, but he was mildly delusional and groggy and slept much more than usual. One morning he burst into my room, sweaty from breaking his fever and smiling devilishly, ready to start some trouble yet again. This revealed another bright side of being sick that follows the law of opposites: health doesn't exist without sickness. It feels so great to be healthy after being sick—we have a new outlook on life, for a few days anyway. His happy outlook lasted for about four days, meaning that neither of us got a nap because he was so grateful!

It is very important to remember the Law of Opposites in every aspect of life. There is no sickness without health, success without failure, like without dislike, good without bad, etc. A failure means only that somewhere success exists, and overwhelm and chaos will usually be followed by higher order and increased coping capabilities. Many sleepless nights and days full of toddler fussiness has resulted in a rather Zen-like mom because it dramatically raised my threshold for such matters. There is always a balance; the fussiness usually results in a longer nap and a happier baby later. Good trade.

Live Outside of the Body

I recall a time on Valentine's Day when I was a kid when my sisters and I received small gifts from our parents and and we were happily playing before dinner time. I sat down at the table to eat when, Whooosshh! My head was ready to fall into my mashed potatoes. I was sick! How is it possible that one minute I was playing, and the next minute I was run down with a fever? My son does the very same thing. He seems to fall ill within just a matter of moments. I thought about this for a while, wondering if illness has a more rapid onset in children than in adults. My conclusion was that children are so unoccupied with their own bodies and preoc- cupied with whatever they are doing that they don't even realize that they are sick until it's something that really requires attention.

I've heard almost every adult that I know say during flu season that they are "coming down with something" for even a few days before they get sick, if they get sick at all. As adults, we seem to fear becoming sick and every sniffle, achy muscle, or scratchy throat is amplified because we pay so much attention to it. Although we are very busy, it is usually with things that we would rather not do; and feeling stressed about that, we focus our attention on what is wrong instead of what is right. Everyone knows that stress inhibits the immune system and produces numerous negative effects on the body. It is just as important to focus on the things that make us happy as it is to eat good food and exercise, maybe even more important. After all, if you are happy, what else do you need?

Live in the Present

My dad always told us, "The things you do today are the memories you will have tomorrow." This is, in fact, a very profound statement, but it's a different language to a teen-ager. What a teenager needs to hear is something like: "If you do stupid teenager stuff like start smoking cigarettes, swearing like a truck driver, and not doing your homework, I'm going to box you up and send you three thousand miles from civilization." Luckily, my son is still a toddler so he only knows how to live in the present. When he is screaming in the car because he has had enough of sitting down, or falls asleep like an angel in my arms at the grocery store, it is because time means nothing to him. Sleeping at night or day or naptime doesn't make any difference. Sleeping when his little body is tired is what matters. He doesn't understand me when I tell him repeatedly that we will be out of the car in ten minutes or that he should eat at a certain time because it is normal lunch or dinner time.

I learned a lot from his living in the present moment. I realized that I do eat when I am not hungry because it is "lunch time," and I make myself go to bed because it is "bed time," even if I lie awake because my body doesn't want to sleep yet. It's the same with working. So much of work time is lost to being unproductive simply because our bodies and brains just aren't feeling it. I have found even writing this very book that if I write only when I feel good about writing, I get more done in about half the time than if I make myself sit down and come up with something.

When people don't want to do something, they procrastinate. It's natural. It would be great if most jobs would allow people to do things at the times that felt right for them—creating highly efficient and productive working environments and maybe even higher quality products—but it is nearly impossible for many businesses to operate in such a manner. Even if it is impossible to accommodate that lifestyle at work, it is possible to live this way in our personal lives. There are always chores that are no fun, like cutting the grass or cleaning, but there is always a better time to do it. The grass can wait until it is sunny and beautiful to cut it, and you have the energy to go outside and at least enjoy the weather while you work. Almost anything can wait until you say, "Okay, I feel like doing something productive. Let's go." Not only will the job get done, but you will feel a lot better about both doing it and the final product.

Living in the present is also important to help us to let go of the past. So often we let our past define who we are. We think things like, "I have always been lazy, so I am a lazy person," or "I never got good grades in school so I am stupid," "or "I have always been overweight so I am a fat person," etc. The problem is that the past is gone. That person is gone forever. If you have ever been something that you didn't like, this is great news! You can choose to become *anything* you want. Your present is only your current reality and it changes every second. From the moment you make a choice about anything, you become that choice and your existence will shift toward that decision. If you change your way of thinking you will also change your way of being. The present is what makes the future. The past doesn't create anything!

Solidarity Prevails!

The slide: a long-beloved piece of playground equipment. Kids around the world whoosh down with the wind in their hair and a smile on their faces. Until one kid decides that he wants to go up the slide instead of down, creating a chain reaction: all of the kids now want to climb up the slide. I personally don't care about this misuse of a slide because I believe that kids go to the park to play, and by gosh if they want to play backwards I don't think that it will affect their growth in any way. I can tell you this, though: many parents can't stand this up-the-slide thing. I guess to some it's as serious an offense as a kick in the crotch or a racial slur. One of two things usually happens at this point: 1.) The parents who don't really care tell their kids not to do it, but they do it anyway and that is that; or 2.) The parents become so incredibly irate at the child that they scold him until they are blue in the face and then carry the child, kicking and screaming, and stuff him into the car to go home for being such a disobedient little schmuck. I'm not qualified to determine which scenario is right or wrong, and it is neither here nor there. I do know that kids will follow other kids and they usually stick together and create the outcome that they want because of their solidarity.

This was a big lesson to me because I must explain that I am a bit of a hermit. I enjoy being alone and I used to ask for the help of others on rare occasions. Now, after seeing the joy that he has experienced playing with others and sharing his toys (most of the time), I decided that it was okay to let others help out and see how greater things can happen if we all come together. I have even seen some "anti-up-the-slide" moms become "it's-not-worth-the-fight" moms and I think it saves them a few hours of turmoil after park sessions. Resistance is rarely a good thing and should be used only in life-threatening situations. I now feel more harmonious with those around me, knowing that we are really all here together, just living, getting by, and trying our best to enjoy as much as we can. Neighbors are meant for sharing cookies with and talking to on a Sunday afternoon, and the guy at the grocery store really does want to help you out to your car in the rain, he's not just asking because he feels the obligation. As long as we are careful with others on the slide I don't think that up or down makes a difference.

$$E = mc^2$$

"Outside!" was my son's first word. He would wake up, watch some cartoons, and then it was time for "outside!" I used to hope that he would one day just give me a few minutes in the morning to wake up before a long stretch of playtime, but now I embrace it. He is the additional jumpstart to my morning coffee. A much-needed one. Mass–energy equivalence states that any object has a certain energy, even when it isn't moving. This just means that we need to find a way to get the energy out! The easiest way to do that is to… Move your butt! Einstein discovered that knocking out that one proton within an atom would create enormous and unstoppable amounts of energy, only to have it used in the wrong way. What a shame. Let's give back to Einstein and find the positive energy within ourselves. Get up and move around, then more energy will follow. My son usually jumps on me to knock out the first proton, which revs me up until at least lunch time. Go nuclear!

Treat the Problem, Not the Symptoms

This morning I was ready to throw in the towel of being a parent, until I found out that this is much different than giving up in a boxing match. My son screamed and fussed all day and all night for a few days and I was at my wits' end. I was worried that he was sick or in pain because of how he just couldn't calm down. It turns out that he did have a big problem. It was me.

Sometime in the few days prior to this incident—and epiphany—my son grew mentally and I didn't notice. I provided him with the same toys and the same television shows, the same trips to the park and the grocery store, the same nap time and the same food. All of these things had been working quite well for us for some time. He would be busy and I would get some things done, then we would play and then nap, and life was good. Today he needed more than that: something new and challenging, and also more attention and teaching from me. I felt awful for missing this, thinking that he was just being a pain in the neck.

Most kids are not a pain in the neck—the problem is just that we don't realize when they need change. Their mental and physical growth accelerate exponentially, requiring parents to reassess and adjust accordingly. Just as plants start out as sprouts and seem to shoot up very quickly, then when they have reached full growth, they just exist, only to change with the seasons. During that sprouting period, the plants are fragile and have greater needs for nourishment and protection than when they are fully grown. Today my son wanted me to read a book with him instead of watching television. He wanted to walk and hold my hand, not be pushed in a stroller, and he would not give up the fight to make me understand that he is evolving into a lovely young boy and that he is not a baby anymore. Before he was able to make me understand his changes and new abilities, I scolded him for being fussy. Now I know better for the next time when he gets so out of sorts that there is more to this guy than what I see now. I need to adjust as well, and find the best ways to accommodate him as he grows, avoiding the trauma and aggravation of these misunderstandings. I wanted to thank him for putting up with me, and more importantly, to teach me that I must also continue to grow.

Many times in life we find that our old system for working through things has worn out and broken down, yet we still continue to try to use it, making for many unhappy and unfulfilled individuals. Though we are like the plants that stop growing physically, we have the capability to grow and change mentally to our greatest desires. Our minds can continue to be the sprout, growing rapidly with new, green, vibrant leaves as often as we want. If we stay in the same place too long, doing the same things that we have always done, we often do become fussy and break down, just as my son did this morning. We need the freshness of new knowledge and experiences to drive us to do better things and to keep on knocking out that next proton, or the energy will stop. We need to continue to find reasons to laugh and feel a sense of accomplishment, giving, and gratitude.

Life can be exactly what we want it to be as long as we stay aware of the ways that we once were and what we should be, and never lose our sense of what we want and what we can achieve. Life is much too short to only go down the slide. We just need to watch out for each other so no one gets hurt.

www.ingramcontent.com/pod-product-compliance
Lightning Source LLC
Chambersburg PA
CBHW032030290526
45786CB00011B/1276